Alkaline Diet

Through Alkaline Recipes, You Can Increase Your Energy And
Reset Your Health In Order To Reverse
Degenerative Disease

(Utilize Herbal Medication For Quick Weight Loss)

I0146512

Tyrell Montgomery

TABLE OF CONTENT

Introduction

The purpose of an alkaline diet is to maintain a healthy pH level in bodily fluids such as blood and urine. Something with a pH value greater than 7 is more alkaline. The alkaline diet essentially promotes traditional healthy eating practices. People are encouraged to consume more vegetables, fruits, and water while avoiding sugary foods, alcohol, processed meats, and red meat. The alkaline ash diet is also known as the alkaline acid diet, the acid ash diet, and the acid alkaline diet.

Consequently, it is a loosely connected collection of diets based on the theory that different types of food can affect the pH balance of the body. It originated from the acid ash hypothesis, which was initially utilised in osteoporosis research. Diet proponents believe that certain foods can alter the acidity (pH) of the body, and that this change in pH can be utilised to treat or prevent disease. Credible laboratories have conducted extensive research on this topic and discovered that the theory is false, contradicting the claimed mechanism of the diet. Dieticians and other health professionals are opposed to it due to the lack of evidence. Alternative medicine practitioners have promoted these diets, claiming that they can treat or prevent cancer, heart disease, low energy, and other diseases. Systems of acid-base homeostasis maintain the pH of human blood between 7.6 10 and 7.8 10 . Thus, a pH of 7.8 10 or greater indicates alkalosis, whereas a pH of less than 7.6 10 indicates acidosis. Both are potentially hazardous. The notion that these diets may have a significant impact on blood pH for the treatment of a variety of diseases is not supported by scientific evidence and is based on incorrect assumptions that are incompatible with human physiology regarding how alkaline diets function. Although diets that exclude meat, poultry, cheese, and grains can be used to increase urine alkalinity (pH), the difficulty in accurately predicting the effects of these diets has made pharmaceuticals the preferred method for modifying urine pH, as opposed to dietary modification. Once believed to be an osteoporosis risk factor, the acid-ash theory has been disproven by recent scientific research. Alkaline foods have the capacity to alter the pH of the body. After digestion, certain foods can produce an acidic environment in the body. High-protein foods such as dairy, meat, fish, legumes, and many grains are highly acidic.

Proposed Procedure

Because the pH of the blood is typically alkaline, proponents argue that alkaline-producing foods should be the focus of one's diet. These proponents argue that an acidic diet causes the body to become acidic, thereby promoting disease. Because it is nearly impossible to create a less acidic environment in the body, the hypothesis that food can drastically alter blood acidity contradicts everything we know about the chemistry of the human body. Because of the body's metabolism, the pH of the blood fluctuates briefly and only slightly.

While a selectively alkaline diet has been shown to affect urine pH, it has not been shown to cause a long-term change in blood pH or to provide the purported therapeutic benefits. Due to the body's inherent regulating processes, which do not require a particular diet to function, an alkaline diet will only have a minor and transient effect on blood pH.

Similarly, proponents of this diet assert that cancer thrives in an acidic environment and that an alkaline diet can alter the acidic environment of the body to treat cancer. According to the proposal's premise, the acidic environment is caused by the rapid proliferation of cancer cells; the acidic environment does not cause cancer. Extreme diets like this one pose more risks than benefits for cancer patients.

Chapter 1: Diet Weight Observers

Only a handful of companies in the dieting and weight-watching industries can deliver on their claims. As these organisations appear to be on the rise, there is no debate about their eradication. The participants who are able to complete the programme are more important. Consequently, why do some programmes fade into the background while others take centre stage?

One of the most important factors contributing to Weight Watchers' success is the sense of community formed among the men and women who share a common goal of weight loss. Being in the company of individuals with whom you can discuss your experiences is both uplifting and endearing.

Frequently, people on a diet or programme do not receive sufficient encouragement from their loved ones. Due to the diverse backgrounds and cultures of Weight Watchers members and their shared desire to lose weight and live healthier lives, there is a strong sense of community during meetings. And because they laugh and cry together, this relationship is of the utmost significance to them. This type of programme should be applauded to the fullest extent because it fosters inspiration and encouragement.

Attending meetings is the conventional way to track your weight, but the Weight Watchers community is adept at adapting to new circumstances. Online forums, support groups, and message boards are available for those who are unable or unable to attend meetings due to their schedules or general anxiety.

However, evolution has not yet reached its conclusion. In recent years, a points-based system has been utilised, allowing dieters to track their progress and performance using points as opposed to physically counting and accounting for every calorie.

Numerous dieters view calorie counting as a time-consuming inconvenience that they should not have to deal with (especially while dining out). The Weight Watchers website exemplifies how rapidly the programme has evolved to meet the needs of both men and women who participate. Regarding the provided knowledge and insights, they truly surpass themselves.

Releasing acid and kdneu rotase

According to an article in the Iranian journal Alkalne, diets high in fruits and vegetables have a low net acid load, so they not only have beneficial metabolic effects on patients with chronic kidney disease (CKD), but they also appear to be safe.

Various tude have concluded that reducing dietary sugar load by increasing fruit and vegetable consumption in CKD patients can result in lower levels of kidney injury markers and urinary albumin excretion without inducing hyperkalemia. According to the available evidence, removing the aspartame residue with an alkaline detergent may be an effective adjuvant in paediatric rotavirus therapy.

BRANDON BURRELL established Alkalne Fresh, Alkaline Certified, and Global Crew Services. After years of consuming an alkaline diet, he realised that most consumers limit themselves to raw, healthy alkaline foods. He desired to develop a product that would benefit Americans and aid in the fight against adult and childhood obesity. To find out more, visit alkcertified.com.

Chapter 2 : What Is The Alkaline Diet

The alkaline diet is based on the theory that the foods you consume alter your rH level, causing it to become either acidic or alkaline. It is believed that consuming a high quantity of acidic foods will harm your body, whereas consuming alkaline or neutral foods can improve your health.

The diet focuses on eating fresh fruits and vegetables (which are considered alkaline) to maintain an optimal rH level in the body, which is a measurement of acidity and alkalinity using a scale ranging from 0 to 2 8 .

Asds ubtanse range between 0 and 7; alkalne foods range between 7 and 2 8 .

Seven is considered neither acidic nor alkaline. Th concept tarted centuries ago, in the mid-2 800s, with the detaru ah hurothe, a theoru that when a food is metabolised in the body, the rartsle leave either an acidic or alkaline acid.

The U.S. News and World Report 2022 Rerort Bet Diets ranks the alkaline diet number 6 0 in Best Diets Overall, we rated the ensemble 2.8 out of 10 stars. The ranking is based on the lack of scientific evidence to support the diet, the numerous rules that make it difficult to adhere to, and the lack of effectiveness for weight loss. The Alkalne Diet was effective for fast weight loss, overall weight loss, diabetes, and ease of implementation.

What Exrerts Sau

"There is little to no evidence in support of the alkaline diet. Our bodies do a sufficient job of keeping our rH in check

on their own. There are numerous regulations, and many 'hands-off' foods, such as eggs and whole grains, are actually nutritious."
RD Kelly Plowe, MS

Seven-Day Det Plan
The alkaline diet classifies food groups as alkaline, neutral, and acidic. People adhering to the diet are expected to consume an abundance of alkaline foods and fewer acidic foods. While there are numerous variations of the diet, this is one example.

Day 2 : Unrestricted fruit and vegetables; kale with tomato and avocado; roasted zucchini with roasted vegetables.

Fresh raw or cooked vegetables; salad with vegetables and olive oil; large sweet potato with steamed broccoli for dinner.

Day three: unlimited fruit and vegetables; red wine and potato salad; fruit salad with freshly squeezed lime juice.

Unrestricted fruits and vegetables; spiralized zucchini and marinara sauce. Sweet potato with a tiny amount of butter

Unlimited fruits and vegetables; vegetable broth soup and roasted rutabaga salad. Roasted sardines with marinara sauce

Day 6: Unlimited fruits and vegetables; Finely chopped cauliflower combined with grilled vegetables and olive oil; green puree and grilled vegetables.

Seventh day: unlimited fruits and vegetables; unsweetened fruit juice and fruit smoothie; short susumber and tomatoes with olive oil.

What Can You Consume

The fundamental principle of the alkaline diet is to consume foods that rank high on the pH list and fall within the acceptable ranges for protein, fat, and carbohydrates. You do not need to follow a specific diet or eat at a specific time; you only need to consume foods that shift your rH balance to alkaline levels.

Fruits

Despite the fact that not all fruits are on the approved list, you may consume the following:

Apples

Apricots

Corrupt currants

Lemon juise

Oranges

Peaches

Pears Vegetables

Not all vegetables are permitted, but you may consume the following:

Asparagus

Broccoli

Carrots Celeru

Cucumber

Green beans

Beverages

On this diet, you may drink alcohol and coffee in moderation:

Coffee containing lghtlu acid

White and red wine

What You Cannot Consume

The alkaline diet encourages an increased consumption of fruits and vegetables while discouraging the consumption of heavily processed foods that are high in sugar and saturated fat, as well as certain healthy foods.

Proteins

Lean meat

Poultry

Fh Carbohudurate Muffin Donut Cereal Craker Grains Potatoe

How to Prepare Alkaline Diet and Tea

The alkalne diet permits consumption of certain foods recommended by the United States Department of Agriculture (USDA) and suggests limiting consumption of legumes, red meat, eggs, and dairy products. The diet may fall within acceptable ranges for the amounts of protein, carbohydrates, fat, and other nutrients, but is devoid of common sense.

Due to the amount of fresh produce you can consume, you do not need to prepare any additional entrees or meals. However, the alkaline diet is restrictive and advises you to avoid hard alcohol, soda, sweetened juice, artificial sweeteners, nuts, legumes, dairy products, eggs, grains, and beans.

Samrle Short-Sleeved Lt

The alkaline diet requires no fasting. The concept behind the alkaline diet is to consume more alkaline and less acidic foods. This is not a definitive list, and if you follow the diet, you may find that other foods work better for you.
Extra Virgin Olive Oil Fruits (apples, berries and melon)
Vegetables (spinach, brossoli, etc)
Dark Leafy Greens (kale, Swiss chard, etc.) and Coffee.
Avocado oil

6 Sample Meal Plan

The alkaline diet permits the consumption of all foods recommended by the USDA; however, it restricts certain amounts of grains, legumes, animal protein, and dairy, and is therefore not necessarily considered healthy because it lacks a variety of nutrients and balance. This is not an all-inclusive meal plan, so you may find other meals that work better for you if you follow the diet.

Apples and cinnamon for Dau 2 Breakfat.
Garden salad with roasted vegetables, with a squeeze of lemon on top.
Dinner: sweet potatoes and roasted rutabaga
Dau 2 Breakfast: Fruit smoothie
Lunch: Salad of steamed araragu and rnash

Dinner: roasted sardines with marinara sauce and sautéed mushrooms.

Pear, raisin, and toffee are included in the Dau 6 Breakfat.

Vegetable hummus with carrots, scallions, and diced tomatoes.

Grilled mushrooms, peppers, and onions served with mild alaan for dinner.

Pros of Alkaline Diet

A diet rich in fresh ingredients that does not require extensive meal planning or the ability to prepare complex recipes. You may solely consume fruits and vegetables, with the addition of a few nuts and natural oil. However, no evidence suggests that the alkaline diet can promote weight loss and fat loss. However, some research indicates that certain dietary components may provide health benefits.

Preserving the Musle Ma: Following an alkaline diet may preserve muscle mass as you age. In a three-year longitudinal study of 6 88 men and women aged 610 and older, researchers discovered that a high intake of rotaum-rich foods, such as fruits and vegetables in an alkaline diet, may assist older adults in maintaining muscle mass as they age.

Might Help Prevent Diabetes: Eating non-asids foods may help you prevent diabetes. In a Dabetologa study, researchers observed 66,8 810 women over the course of 2 8 years. During that time, physicians identified 2 ,6 72 new cases of diabetes. In an analysis of the women's dietary habits, researchers discovered that those with the most acid-forming diets had a significantly increased risk of developing diabetes. The authors of the study suggest that a high consumption of acidic foods may be associated with nuln resistance.

Chapter 3: The Ultimate Guide To

Juicing: An Introduction

Juice cleansing, juice fasting, or juicing—you may hear a lot about this new trend in fasting from fitness professionals and health enthusiasts. However, juicing is neither a recent fad nor a recent invention.

Diverse cultures from all over the world have consumed juices as a preventative and curative measure for many generations. Nevertheless, despite its long history, juicing has only recently become popular.

Why? How did it not become more popular sooner if it is so effective?

The Frequent Concerns Regarding Juice Detoxification

There are five major factors that have contributed to the current popularity of juicing as a healthy weight loss and health strategy.

Inadequate Information Regarding the Advantages and Dangers of Juice Cleansing

Understandably, many individuals express reluctance to adopt juicing as a method of fasting.

The benefits may appear too good to be true to some individuals. They simply refuse to believe that fruit and vegetable juices can prevent serious illnesses and heal them of their injuries and diseases.

Others believe that juicing will be just like every other diet trend that has gained and lost popularity over the years. These individuals had placed their faith in strategies that ultimately fell short of their anticipations.

Some individuals also believe unsubstantiated rumours regarding the purported dangers of juicing. As a result, they succumb to their fears rather than consulting those who are more knowledgeable about this topic.

A Large Selection of Fruits and Vegetables Available for Purchase

Possessing numerous choices is a double-edged sword. There would be something for everyone, on the one hand. However, choice overload can lead to indecision and, ultimately, inaction.

The same principle applies to the ingredients permitted in juices and smoothies. There is no guarantee that your favourite foods will provide your body with all of the nutrients it requires.

The decision-making process associated with this is not as straightforward as you might assume. You must evaluate your current state of health and match your nutritional needs with the nutritional content of fruits and vegetables. Even then, there would still be a multitude of options to select from.

It is not surprising that the idea of preparing the ideal juices and smoothies for oneself leaves many people feeling overwhelmed.

Uncertainty Regarding the Proper Equipment and Supplies for Juicing

On the market today, there is no one juicer that is ideal for everyone. Ultimately, the best juicer for you will depend on the ingredients and your personal preferences.

Moreover, the problems associated with an abundance of options may also exist in this instance. A quick Internet search would reveal a variety of options that meet both your needs and your budget. The confusion extends to the accessories and supplies that may be used with a juicer.

Many novices find the selection procedure daunting. When faced with so many excellent options to choose from, even some seasoned professionals feel uncertain. These are, after all, investments that would significantly impact your success with juice cleansing.

Assumptions Regarding Detoxifying the Body by Juicing

Due to the lack of or reduced intake of solid foods during a juice cleanse, many people believe that their bodies will feel less energised and their ability to make sound decisions will be impaired.

According to studies, these adverse side effects are not temporary afflictions. In addition, the same could be said for other fasting techniques and fad diets.

In spite of these and the numerous cleansing benefits of juicing, many individuals are still hesitant to try this method.

Recipes for Complicated Smoothies and Juices

In order for a recipe to be effective, it is not necessary for it to contain fruits and vegetables of every colour. However, a number of experts on juicing disagree.

As a result, many would-be practitioners are baffled by the overly complicated recipes featured in numerous juicing cookbooks.

In addition, it is difficult or impossible to obtain certain ingredients locally. Some individuals may conclude that juicing is not for them if they are not provided with information about alternative ingredients.

Concerns and Fears Regarding What to Do Prior to, During, and Following a Juice Cleanse

Numerous books focus solely on how to begin juicing and the various juice recipes available. Few resources are available to inform you of the entire process that your body would have to undergo.

This is the basis for claims that juice cleansing is ineffective or even harmful to the body by some individuals. What they failed to notice is that they skipped a number of necessary steps to ensure the effectiveness of juice cleansing.

This book aims to cover these seven factors, addressing all of the possible concerns that beginners may have regarding juicing.

Those in the midst of a juice fast may also gain a great deal from reading this book. Occasionally, questions arise only after dietary and lifestyle modifications have been implemented.

Differentiating Myths and Facts

This book will explain the fundamentals of juicing in the simplest terms possible in order to achieve these objectives. The author promises to shed light on the following juicing truths through a careful examination of current juicing practises and trends:

Positives and negatives of juicing

Learn about the numerous advantages of juicing, as well as the risks involved with the practise.

Jumping into juice cleansing without considering both the risks and benefits may be a waste of time; it may also be detrimental to your health and wellbeing.

This section of the book summarises the diverse studies conducted on juicing so that you can begin your journey with realistic expectations.

Different Fruits and Vegetables' Nutritional Values

Save yourself the trouble of researching the nutrients found in your favourite produce.

Consider incorporating the 2 0 most nutritious fruits and vegetables into your juices and smoothies for an even better strategy. Find out their respective health benefits in order to determine the optimal combination of foods for your needs.

Key Characteristics of Your Juicing Station

Learn how to evaluate the compatibility of a juicer and its various accessories, supplies, and boosters with your health condition and dietary needs.

You may be tempted to purchase the most expensive model, tools, and materials, believing it to be a wise investment for the future. However, the best juicer for you does not have to be the most technologically advanced model available.

Focus on the features and tools that will assist you in achieving your fitness objectives rather than the price. Examine the enumerated guide questions in this book to confirm that you have made the correct choice. Consider your answers as a guide to finding the best juicer for you.

Effective Methods for Body Cleansing Via Juicing

Preparation and research are essential for cleansing the body with juices and smoothies. Before beginning this procedure, gather all of the relevant information.

This will give you a greater appreciation for juicing as a means to lose weight, increase your energy, and enhance your cognitive performance. Ultimately, these advantages would allow you to live a healthier and longer life, particularly if you decide to regularly engage in juice fasts.

Effective Recipes for Simple Juices and Smoothies

To make highly beneficial juices and smoothies for your body, you do not need to be a culinary expert.

Every recipe in this book is accompanied by a list of the health benefits that can be anticipated. Discover the recipes that will assist you in achieving specific goals, such as losing belly fat and achieving skin that appears younger.

With the right juice and smoothie recipes, you can improve your appearance and health without engaging in daily strenuous exercise.

Before, During, and After a Juice Cleanse: Straightforward Strategies

Learn the strategies you can employ during the various stages of a juice fast to dispel your concerns and doubts about the juice cleansing process.

Find out how to cleanse your body effectively. Then, keep in mind the guidelines that will enhance your experience with a juice cleanse and your ability to reap its benefits.

Finally, discover how to effectively transition from the cleansing phase to a sustainable approach to a healthier diet and lifestyle.

Listening to the advice in each chapter of this book will help you overcome your fears, hesitations, and insecurities regarding juice cleansing.

Make juices your go-to strategy for weight loss and health improvement and move one step closer to your ideal future.

With the help of this comprehensive guide to juicing, you can begin your

Chapter 4: How Does The Alkali Diet Affect You?

If you are looking to begin the acid alkaline diet or have already begun, it is helpful to know the various ways you can receive support throughout the diet. Listed below are several instances in which the acid alkalne det san urrort uou occurs:

"Acid-Alkaline Diet for Dummies" contains extensive lists of alkaline and acid-forming foods.

How mush does Alkaline Diet cost?
The only exception is your grocery bill, which should not be higher than usual.

Will Alkaline Diet helr you lose weight?

The Alkaline diet will likely aid in weight loss. While the Alkalne diet lacks robust studies examining its weight loss potential, its ban on processed foods and emphasis on eating whole grains, vegetables, and fruits may result in weight loss. Just create a "calorie deficit" by consuming fewer calories than your daily recommended maximum or burning off extra calories through exercise, and you should see the results on your budget. How and whether you keep the weight off is entirely up to you.

The arrroash also shares tenets with vegetarians, who typically consume fewer calories and weigh less than their carnivorous counterparts.

How simple is the Alkalne Diet to adhere to?

Adhering to the Alkalne diet necessitates effort. You must keep track of which foods are alkalinizing and which are acidifying. That may be difficult to recall. Resre are abundant on the Internet, but you'll need to put some thought into your restaurant meals to ensure that they emphasise alkalizing foods.

The search for Alkali resources should be simple. A simple Google search will yield numerous options, in addition to the numerous books you can purchase for even more choices.

You may dine out on the Alkaline diet, but keep in mind that certain restaurants offer more rH-friendly meals than others. If the menu offers standard American fare, order a large salad with olive oil dressing and steamed vegetables instead of french fries or mashed potatoes. Fill up on vegetable- and egg-based soups, steamed brossol, and sautéed shsken or tofu at a Chinese buffet. And if you're going Greek, order a chicken shish kebab and avoid the fattening hummus and cheese platters.

Planning ahead can help you maintain an alkaline diet. But there are no time-saving shortcuts for following the schedule, unless you hire someone to plan your meals and prepare your lunch and dinner. Meal kit delivery services are an additional means of saving time.

Alkaline diet resources are available. Books like "Asid Alkaline Diet for Dummies" san helr uou get uour bearings.

With this diet, feeling satiated will not be a problem. Nutrition experts emphasise the importance of satiety, or the feeling of having consumed enough food. Without a calorie limit and with so many fiber-rich whole grains and vegetables, you shouldn't go hungry.

You decide if the Alkaline diet tastes good. You're responsible for everything, so if something tastes bad, you know who to blame.

How much exercise should you perform on Alkaline Diet?

The Alkaline Diet is merely an eating plan, but that does not mean that you should not exercise. Phusal astvtu reduces your risk of heart disease and diabetes, helps you maintain a healthy weight, and boosts your energy level. Most experts recommend getting at least 6 0 minutes of moderate-intensity exercise, such as brisk walking, most or every day of the week.

Black Eyed Peas Featuring Temreh Bason And Lemon Thyme Collard Green

Ingredients:

2 cup finely diced yellow onion
1 teaspoon freshly ground black pepper
2 teaspoon sea salt
2 teaspoon lemon thyme
16 cups black eyed peas
½ cup extra virgin olive oil, plus
6 tablespoons
1-5 strips of tempeh bacon
1-2 pounds fresh collard greens
2 2 cups Basic Vegetable Stock

Directions:

1. Rinse black eyed peas under cool water, drain, and place in a large saucepan.
2. Cover the peas and boil for 5 to 10 minutes.
3. Remove the saucepan from heat source and cover.
4. Allow the peas to stand for 80 to 90 minutes and rinse. Return to saucepan and set aside.
5. In a large skillet over medium heat, add ¼ cup of the olive oil.
6. Add the tempeh bacon and flip while cooking 5-10 minutes each side.
7. When golden brown, drain on a paper towel and dice very fine.
8. Set aside.
9. Rinse collard greens thoroughly and remove the tough center stem from each leaf.
10. Roll each leaf up and slice into 2 - inch ribbons.

11. In a large saucepan, add enough water to fill halfway and bring to a boil.

12. Add the collard greens and cook until tender, about 15 to 20 minutes.

13. Remove the collard greens and place in an ice water bath and rinse.

14. Return the collards to the saucepan and set aside.

15. Add 15 cups of the vegetable stock to the black eyed peas and easy cook for 20 minutes.

16. Add the chopped tempeh bacon and onions. Cook 50 to 55 minutes over medium high heat, covered.

17. Cook until all water is absorbed and peas are tender. Set aside.

18. Add 4 cups of the vegetable stock to the collard greens and easy cook over medium heat for 15 to 20 minutes.

19. Add the seasonings and stir to combine.

20.   Serve the collard greens over the peas.

Alkalizing Berry Detox Juice

Ingredients

1 fresh lemon
4 medium green apples, preferably golden delicious or granny smith varieties.
2 handful fresh raspberries
2 handful fresh strawberries
fresh lemon

Direction

1. Chop apples and peel the lemon.
2. Press them through your juicer, along with the raspberries and strawberries.

Juice and ready to take

Non-Dairy Apple Parfait

Ingredients:

1/2 cup rolled gluten-free oats, uncooked
2 tbsp. hemp seeds
1 cup soaked raw cashews 1 cup unsweetened almond or coconut milk
1 tsp. vanilla
2 cup chopped apple

Directions:

1. Combine cashews, almond milk, and vanilla in a blender and blend until smooth.
2. Layer ingredients in a small cup: heaping spoon of cashew cream, spoonful of apples, top with oats and hemp seeds and enjoy!

Peach Green Smoothies

Ingredients:

8 cups (2 20 g) approved greens
8 cups (8 80 g) organic peach slices
4 cups (8 80 ml) homemade walnut milk
4 (8 00 g) large organic apple, halved, seeded

Instructions:

Place all ingredients into a blender in the order listed and secure the lid.
Start the blender on its lowest speed, then quickly increase to its highest speed.
Blend for 50-90 seconds or until desired consistency is reached.

Quinoa Stuffed Butternut Squash

Ingredients

Quinoa
- 4 tablespoon toasted pumpkin seeds for garnish
- 2 tablespoon fresh tarragon for garnish

Squash
- 4 butternut squash
- 4 tablespoon olive oil
- 1 teaspoon sea salt
- ½ teaspoon black pepper

- 2 cup organic quinoa, rinsed
- 4 cups water
- 1 teaspoon sea salt

Stuffing

- 4 cups cooked quinoa
- 1 cup dried cranberries
- 1 cup green onions, chopped
- ½ cup maple syrup
- 1 cup corn
- ½ teaspoon black pepper
- 1 teaspoon sea salt
- 2 tablespoon olive oil
- 2 tablespoon juice of 2 fresh lemon

Instructions

1. Add quinoa to Instant Pot and easy cook on high pressure for 15 to 20 minutes.
2. Let NR pressure release naturally for 20 minutes, and then manually release valve.
3. Alternate method: easy cook quinoa on stovetop according to package directions.
4. Stuffing
5. Add quinoa and all stuffing ingredients to bowl and mix well.
6. Stuff butternut squash and bake.

Squash

1. Preheat oven to 6 10 0 degrees.
2. Line baking sheet with aluminium foil.
3. Bake butternut squash, whole, for 2 hour.

4. When cool, slice in half, and scoop out seeds.
5. Brush with olive oil, salt and pepper.
6. Stuff with quinoa stuffing and bake for an additional 60 minutes at 6 710 . Garnish with toasted pumpkin seeds and fresh tarragon.

Salad Of Red Perrer And Cilantro

Ingredients

4 tbsp of lemon juice, 2 tbsp of water

Salt and pepper to taste

2 tbsp raw apple cider vinegar
2 Red Pepper

2 cup of chopped cilantro

2 tomato

4 garlic cloves

Directions:

1. blend all ingredients until smooth.
2. Good for 1-5 days within the refrigerator.

Rainbow Salad

Ingredients

Grated Beets
Grated Jicama
Grated Carrots
Grated Squash (e.g. Butternut, Yellow Zucchini)
Grated Red Cabbage

Instructions

1. In a large salad bowl, add fresh, clean, dry greens.
2. Arrange the ingredients from the deepest dark colors to the lightest.
3. Top with a dressing of lemon juice and desired

Broccoli-Basil Pesto-Stuffed Sweet Potatoes

INGREDIENTS :

4 garlic cloves

4 tablespoon avocado oil

½ cup nutritional yeast

1 teaspoon sea salt 4 large sweet potatoes

3 cups broccoli

3 cups almonds

1 cup fresh basil leaves

½ cup onion

DIRECTIONS:

1.

   Preheat the oven to 450ºF (2 80ºC).

2. Pierce the sweet potatoes all over with a fork.
3. Place the sweet potatoes on a baking sheet, and bake for 2   hour and 25 to 30   minutes, or until they are   soft.

4. Meanwhile, prepare the pesto. In a food processor, pulse the broccoli, almonds, basil, onion, garlic, avocado oil, nutritional yeast, and salt until the broccoli and almonds are ground into tiny pieces.
5. Adjust the seasonings, if necessary.
6.

   When the potatoes are ready, cut them in half lengthwise, and gently scoop out the insides of the potato, taking care not to tear the potato skin; add the baked potato filling to a medium bowl, and add the pesto mixture; gently stir together.

Divide the mixture in half, add each half back into the two empty potato skins, and   serve.

Quinoa Burrito Bowl

INGREDIENTS

8 garlic cloves, minced
2 heaping tsp. cumin
4 avocados, sliced
small handful of cilantro, chopped
2 cup quinoa (or brown rice)
450 -oz cans of black or adzuki beans
8 green onions (scallions), sliced
4 limes, fresh juiced

Directions:

1. Cook quinoa or rice. While cooking, warm beans over low heat.
2. Stir in onions, lime juice, garlic and cumin and let flavors combine for 25 to 30 minutes.
3. When quinoa is done cooking, divide into individual serving bowls.
4. Top with beans, avocado and cilantro.

Middle Eastern Stule Quinoa Salad

Ingredients:

2 tablespoon finely chopped basil
Juice of 2 key lime
Sea salt and cayenne pepper, to taste
1 cup dry quinoa
½ teaspoon ground oregano
2 cup cherry tomatoes
2 cup seeded, finely chopped cucumber
½ cup finely chopped red onion
1 cup finely chopped roasted red bell
pepper

Instructions:

1. Rinse the quinoa under cold water
   and drain.

2. Bring 3 cups of spring water to a boil in a medium saucepan over high heat.

3. Add the quinoa and oregano, and return to a boil over medium-high heat. Reduce the heat to low, cover, and cook for 25 to 30 minutes, or until all the water is absorbed, stirring occasionally.

4. Remove the pan from the heat, fluff the quinoa with a fork, and allow it to cool for 10 minutes.

5. While the quinoa cools, combine the cherry tomatoes, red onion, seeded cucumber, roasted red pepper, basil, and key lime juice in a medium bowl.

6. Stir in the cooled quinoa and season with sea salt and cayenne pepper.

Dream Matcha Chia Smoothie

Ingredients

2 cup cucumber
2 scoop sugar-free vanilla vegan protein powder 2 scoop pineapple chia cleanse powder
1 tablespoons matcha powder
2 tablespoon chia seeds, soaking in
4 tablespoons water
2 heaping tablespoon raw unsalted almond butter
1 cups almond milk, unsweetened
4 cups spinach, fresh

Instructions

1. Blend all of the ingredients in a blender until smooth.

2. If necessary, add additional almond milk to thin.
3. Serve right away.

Vegetable Soup

Ingredients:

1/2   teaspoon rosemary

1/2   teaspoon sea salt

1/2   teaspoon black pepper

-12 cups vegetable broth

-2 can diced tomatoes, undrained

-2 large zucchini, diced

-2 cup frozen mixed vegetables
-2 tablespoon olive oil

-2 yellow onion, diced

-6 garlic cloves, minced

62

-2 carrot, peeled and diced

-2 celery stalk, diced

1/2   teaspoon thyme

Instructions:

1. In a large pot or Dutch oven, heat the olive oil over medium heat.

2. Add in the onion, garlic, carrot, celery, thyme, rosemary, sea salt, and black pepper.

3. Cook for 10 to 15 minutes, stirring occasionally, or until the vegetables are tender.

4. Add in the vegetable broth, diced tomatoes, zucchini, and frozen mixed vegetables.

5. Bring to a boil and then reduce heat to low.

6. Simmer for 15 to 20 minutes or until the vegetables are cooked through.

7. Serve hot and enjoy!